The Bankrupt Australian Health System

Dr David A Corbett

Published in Australia by Corvus Publishing
Street: 4/1 Violet St ESSENDON, 3040
Email: dcorbett@westnet.com.au
Website: dcorbett.com.au

First published in Australia 2014
Copyright © Dr David A Corbett 2013
Cover design, John Lowe
Typesetting: Felicity Gilbert

National Library of Australia Cataloguing-in-Publication entry
Author: Corbett, David A. (David Albert), 1940- author.
Title: The bankrupt Australian health system / David A Corbett.
ISBN: 9780992414412 (paperback)
Notes: Includes index.

Subjects: Medical policy--Australia.
Health planning--Australia.
Public health--Australia.
Medical care--Australia.

Dewey Number: 362.10994

Disclaimer
All care has been taken in the preparation of the information herein, but no
responsibility can be accepted by the publisher or author for any damages
resulting from the misinterpretation of this work. All contact details given in
this book were current at the time of publication, but are subject to change.

The advice given in this book is based on the experience of the individuals.
Professionals should be consulted for individual problems. The author and
publisher shall not be responsible for any person with regard to any loss or
damage caused directly or indirectly by the information in this book.

By the same author
The Lies of the Land
Important Principles of Anaesthesia
The Fantasies of Modern Physics

ABOUT THE AUTHOR

David Corbett graduated in Medicine from Melbourne University in 1964. He subsequently trained as a specialist Anaesthetist. He has spent one year in the United States, one year in Saudi Arabia and many years in city and rural hospitals in Australia in that specialty.

He has also gained qualifications in accounting, finance and investment and has a diploma from the Institute of Company Directors. He has a continued interest in mathematics and physics as well as studying Electronic engineering for four years part time. He was also a Councillor on the Essendon City Council for three years.

THIS BOOK IS DEDICATED

To my younger colleagues
…. whose talents are being so cruelly wasted

and

To my country
…. which deserves so much better

CONT|ENTS

PRE|FACE

Australia has been lumbered with an overly expensive health system, and one that is unsustainable. The system was badly conceived and only introduced to gain political votes. The chickens are now coming home to roost, with an ineffective distribution of medical personnel, poor service and an unbearable cost to the government. There are simple answers to the problem, but politicians must face reality. They must admit that the system is flawed and revert to sensible economic management.

INTRO|DUCTION

The health system in Australia is reaching crisis point. Planning for the future is in chaos, there will soon be an over-supply of nurses and doctors, and the cost of health care is exploding.

Australia has a high concentration of doctors in city areas and insufficient numbers in rural areas. Because of the lack of locally trained doctors, up to 40% of our medical workforce is foreign-trained and these foreign graduates mainly staff our country hospitals.

The waiting lists for elective surgery are getting longer every year. In 2012, patient waiting times in Victoria for the two commonest surgical specialties were 41–46 days (for general surgery) and 63–76 days (for orthopedic surgery). The proportion of those waiting over a year for elective surgery in those two specialties was in excess of 2.0% and 4.4% respectively.

We have ambulances lining up outside hospitals—sometimes up to seven deep—because there are not enough medical staff to keep the emergency departments clear. The time ambulances spend waiting to off-load patients is known as "ramping". Between 1st January and 30th June

2012, ambulances wasted a total of 3,975 hours ramping at just one major Melbourne hospital.

Patients sometimes lie on gurneys in emergency departments for more than 24 hours before being admitted to a hospital bed.

When people look at the Australian health system, they see it to be dysfunctional and believe that this is due to a lack of funding. But is funding the real problem? Is there any country that provides comparable or better health care at a cheaper rate? In fact, to our shame, there is. Consider table 1 below and note the performance of Cuba.

Table 1: Medical resources, costs, and outcomes: 2012

Measure	Australia	USA	Cuba
Life expectancy at birth	81	78	79
Child (<5) mortality/1000 of population	5	8	5
Health expenditure:			
U.S. $ per capita	3,484	7,960	478
% of GDP	8.7	17.6	5.91
Doctors/1000 population	2.50	2.30	5.91

Source: World Health Organization

Despite USA embargoes against imports of drugs and equipment, Cuba seems to be out-performing Australia (and the USA) on a number of important measures. Some further interesting facts about the Cuban health system are as follows:

- Life expectancy in Cuba is 79 years, one of the highest in the region.

- The Cuban mortality rate is the third lowest in the world.

- On a per capita basis, the prevalence of AIDS is only one sixth that of the US.

- In 1999, Cuba had one doctor for every 170 people.

- Cuba is presently training about 8 medical undergraduates from the USA who cannot afford to pay for training in their own country.

What? Cuba spends only $478 per person on health and yet can train almost 6 physicians per 1000 of population when Australia spends $3,484 and can only train 1.5? Fidel Castro rubbed further salt into the wound by offering to send 1,500 physicians to the USA to help after Hurricane Katrina devastated New Orleans.

Something here just doesn't add up.

In Australia, we have a system which has grown like Topsy, with the result that there is an enormous wastage of health funds. Funds are being diverted to unnecessary bureaucracy and to purposes totally unrelated to health care.

In order to understand how to deal with these problems, we need to understand what forces exist, how they developed and how they need to be changed in order to correct the present mess.

1 | N A T I O N A L
       H E A L T H
       S Y S T E M S

Following the Second World War, Britain introduced a national health system. Initially, this service—in place by 1948—was free at point-of-service and funded by general taxation.

After the introduction of the British system, tentative efforts were made to introduce something similar in Australia. However, resistance by the medical profession stalled the introduction of an Australian system until 1973. The decline of standards of patient care in England due to its national health system provided good evidence that the reticence of Australian doctors was justified. By 1970, other countries—such as Sweden and Canada—had introduced national health systems that were also showing signs of trouble.

The American philosopher George Santayana once stated that those who will not learn the lessons of history are condemned to repeat it. The problem is that the real lessons of history are never taught. Dates and bare facts might get taught, but not the reasons why events occur. For example, we are taught that in 1066 William the Conqueror invaded England, but why did he do it?

If we analyzed history and learned the obvious consequences of actions, we would make fewer mistakes than we presently do. Because we rarely consider in detail what will happen if we perform a given act, we tend to make the same dumb mistakes time and time again.

The fact that no lessons are learned from history has often been parodied as *The only lesson to be learned from history is that no-one ever learns anything from history.*

Thus it should come as no surprise to learn that those who introduced the national health system in Australia never took note of the problems that were obvious in comparable overseas systems.

The Australian national health push was set rolling by Graeme Perkin, the editor of *The Age* newspaper in Melbourne. In the mid-1960s, he published a three-part article over three consecutive Saturdays entitled "Medicine in the Market Place". The article queried whether doctors were dedicated to the treatment of patients or whether their primary interest was the acquisition of wealth. His passion was ignited by a personal experience he had had with the treatment of his father.

At this time, the Australian Labor Party had been in opposition for about two decades and was especially keen to regain power. The introduction of a national health scheme seemed like a good idea at the time as it had wide public support and thus was a potential vote winner.

But the politicians never considered the repercussions of the particular national health scheme they were proposing. First, the cost of the scheme was bound to become exponentially expensive. Second, the introduction of the scheme would only win votes on one occasion. At the next election, voters would be looking to be plied with a fresh set of goodies.

Doctors warned of three main dangers with the proposed scheme:

- A scheme in which the patient paid nothing was bound to be over-used by patients.

- A scheme which cost the patient nothing would lead to doctors over-servicing.

- Giving every citizen an open check book would become prohibitively expensive for the government.

These warnings were ignored and Medibank—the name given to the national health service—was introduced. It was claimed to be a great political reform, and it was not to be thwarted by the concerns of doctors. Whenever these concerns were aired, the Labor Party and the press embarked on a vilification campaign against doctors. Doctors were labeled "greedy bastards" and their attempt to sabotage the introduction of such an illustrious scheme was deemed to be born of mere self-interest.

This vilification led to violence. The walls of some doctors' surgeries were daubed with slogans such as "The AMA makes me sick" and some doctors were run off the road as they drove along. (In those days, doctors who were members of the Australian Medical Association (AMA) affixed the symbol of the Cross of Malta to their cars. They don't do that anymore.) As a result of this intimidation and violence, many doctors took self-defense courses.

The bitterness and lack of trust whipped up by the government at the time continues to color the relationship between government and the medical profession. Doctors today still have no trust and little respect for government, and this antagonism will not be resolved easily. But it must eventually be resolved if our health system is to become sustainable.

On gaining government, the Labor Party introduced a bill to the Federal Parliament that was subsequently called the *Health Insurance Act 1973* (also known as the *Medibank Act*). The Act was strongly opposed by the opposition parties and required a double dissolution of the Federal Government to enact it. A double dissolution forces a new election for all seats in the Senate and the House of Representatives. The bills that caused the double dissolution are then voted on by a joint sitting of both houses of parliament: the Senate and the House of Representatives. When the bill to introduce a national health scheme was introduced to the joint sitting, it was passed.

As the *Health Insurance Act* created a system whereby every citizen had access to medical care at no direct cost to themselves, the system was bound to become prohibitively expensive, and for three main reasons:

1. *Every citizen had basically been given an open check book with which to write unlimited checks on the government.*

If a government introduces such a system and the government has to pay the real cost while the user pays nothing, it follows that the government must eventually go bankrupt.

The problem for government is that it is always hard to withdraw a concession that people have come to expect. Money given to people with trivial complaints is obviously money that cannot be used for more important purposes, such as providing new hips and knees to those whose lives continue to be intolerable without them.

But there are more votes in people with coughs and colds than there are in people requiring new hips, and the government was more interested in votes and redistribution of wealth than in prudent economic management.

2. *As new medical techniques requiring new equipment are invented, there must be an increase in costs.*

A notable example of this is endoscopy, a technique unknown prior to the introduction of Medibank. Another example is gastroscopy. Few gastroscopies were performed before Medibank, but with the advent of more sophisticated equipment, some surgeons are now performing ten or more per week. At a cost exceeding $150 per procedure, this adds $1500 per operating surgeon per week to the cost of Medicare.

3. *Over-servicing by doctors.*

As there was no incentive for doctors to rein in costs, the opportunity arose to provide medical services that were not completely necessary but could be excused on the grounds that they were important for a patient's welfare. This became worse as litigation against doctors increased. To protect themselves, doctors ordered a multitude of tests in order to avoid any accusation that they were not thorough enough.

When the chickens came home to roost—and virtually every problem about which doctors had warned came to pass—doctors were no longer accused only of being "greedy bastards". They were now blamed for everything that was going wrong.

The outcome was that doctors ceased giving suggestions as to how the service might be improved (not that they were ever encouraged to do so). The attitude of the profession became: "OK, you do it your way and we'll look after ourselves". The schism produced by the political vilification has resulted in a lack of medical input into national health strategy. This is costing the government, and ultimately the public, an enormous amount of public money.

Not all doctors were opposed to the introduction of Medibank. As it has turned out, Medibank—and Medicare as it was later called—has been a financial bonanza to the profession. Medicare guarantees the incomes of all doctors and this income can easily be expanded by any doctor to meet their personal financial needs. If the purpose of Medibank was to limit the income of doctors, it has failed spectacularly. Most doctors tripled their incomes within two years. Doctors were soon buying Rolls Royces at a prodigious rate and overseas trips were the order of the day. One day, I noted a consultant doctor arriving at the hospital in a medium-priced Ford car. When I asked what had become of his Rolls Royce, he told me that he had sold it because he was fed up being abused by people he didn't even know.

The concept of a national health scheme is not inherently wrong, but the way it was introduced was far from clever. It led to a breakdown of trust between doctors and government, and many doctors came to adopt the attitude of "every one for themselves". Rectifying the problems will require, at the very least, the removal of a host of politically appointed health bureaucrats who presently siphon enormous amounts of money out of the system without providing any demonstrable value in return.

For some reason the introduction of a national health system in Australia has been hailed as a great reform. However, it has become the major cause of the damage done to the Australian health care system and is gradually destroying the Australian economy.

Probably the greatest exploiter of the weaknesses of the Australian national health system was a person we shall call Ged (not his real name). Ged's wholly legal exploitation was breathtaking, surpassing the efforts of many others who tried a similar approach but ended their careers in suicide. As Ged sallied forth he left in his wake a Medicare financial system that looked for all the world like a field of recently harvested wheat. His generous return of largesse to the community ranged from the establishment of luxury medical centers to the support of a football team which brought great joy to those less fortunate north of the Victorian border. Politicians agreed that the Australian community deserved such opulence and praised his efforts. They had to, of course, because Ged was doing everything by the book. But doing everything by the book does not necessarily lead to the books being balanced at the end of the day. Eventually, Ged, somewhat akin to his football team, ceased to kick goals and the authorities began to take their revenge. This may have been because they resented doctors sniggering at them or because Ged had had the audacity to reveal their inordinate stupidity. Who knows?

Private health insurance ——————————

A particularly deceptive method used by government to contain the cost of health care has been its support for private health insurance. Government encourages people to take out private health insurance and even provides concessions to those who do and penalties to those who don't.

Most people take out private health insurance in the belief that they might otherwise not get medical treatment in an emergency. Wrong! If you really need urgent treatment, you will get it. Doctors just can't help themselves. Of course, if the treatment is not urgent, you may have to wait some time—often considerable time—if you are not insured.

The government encourages private insurance because it shifts a considerable cost burden from itself on to the community in general. That is, the privately insured person is paying what amounts to an extra tax for the privilege of being responsible for his or her own health.

Government has introduced community rating. This means that all insured people pay the same premium for insurance *regardless of risk*. (Traditionally, insurance premiums are rated according to risk: if there is a high risk that a claim will be made, the premium will be higher than if there is a low risk.) Now, approximately 12% of those over 65 years of age have private health insurance. This figure has remained reasonably constant over the decades. But for every dollar the over-65s contribute to the pool of medical funds, they take out over six dollars. This is not surprising as the over-65s have a greater risk of illness and require more medical interventions than younger age groups. But guess who is paying the extra five or so dollars? Because of community rating it is the under-65s. Moreover, the under-65s are financially penalized if they do not have private health insurance. But enforcing private health insurance on the under-65s at the risk of penalty amounts to extortion.

If enough people leave private health insurance, the government will be forced to remove the extortionate community rating and let insurance companies insure according to risk. That is, you will now be insuring yourself and not every other medical cripple and his dog.

Here's an idea: use the money you currently pay for medical insurance to pay off your house. Arrange with your bank to allow the equity you have in your house to be used as a line of credit. If you need to pay private fees to get a quick operation, the chances are that you will be much further ahead with your house mortgage than you would otherwise be. In fact, the chances are that you will never need an urgent private operation, and thus you will be in clover, having paid off your house much earlier than you expected. If you don't have a mortgage, put the money aside and save up for one.

To get riskier patients into the private sector, the government has:

- rebated 30% of the private premium

- imposed a levy on those not privately insured and

- enforced community rating on insurers, with the result that privately insured people help to pay for those that the government should be paying for.

2 | P O L I T I C S

To understand politics one must learn to interpret words in ways other than their literal meaning. Whenever a politician talks of introducing *reform*, realize that this is a euphemism for *cock-up*. Notable examples include health system reform (cock-up) and education reform (cock-up).

Cock-ups might not be inevitable, but the pattern throughout history strongly suggests that they are. There is one over-riding reason why cock-ups occur: politicians never consider in detail the consequences of the actions they take. (In fairness, this phenomenon is not restricted to politicians. Most of us act first and think of the consequences later.)

Isaac Newton stated a universal law when he said that every action has an equal and opposite reaction. If you want to paint your house yellow, your neighbour will inevitably complain that such an action depreciates the value of their property. And every boxer knows that whenever thy make an aggressive movement, that movement also opens them up to attack. A boxer who does not realize this ends up on the canvas.

The message is simple: whenever an action is

contemplated, one must always consider the obvious response (reaction) to that action. Any great reform a government wishes to introduce will cause some undesirable effects and inconvenience someone. All the government has to do is think of what those effects are likely to be and either offset them or not proceed with the reform. However, as many political actions are meant to win votes or to be monuments to a particular politician, the initial action is usually more important than the consequences.

When there is interference with the trajectory of any economy, the response is never immediate. Let us say that the economy is trending downwards and politicians make a corrective change. The economy does not immediately bend sharply upwards. What happens is that there is a gradual levelling out and then a reversal towards growth. This is known as the *J-curve effect*. A similar effect occurs when the economy is trending upward and politicians stab it in the back. The curve then looks more like an inverted umbrella handle. The transition in either case is one to an initial levelling followed by a reversal of the trajectory.

The *Health Insurance Act* was purely a political device to gain votes. The desire to win votes was so strong that it suppressed any serious consideration of the *Act's* likely consequences. But the damage caused by its introduction did not become obvious immediately. Indeed, papering-over the problems by people of good will meant that the enormity of the damage caused by the *Health Insurance Act* took a long time to become apparent: as many as three decades, in fact.

In the 1990s, the government noticed that the cost of the health system was blowing out. On the basis that doctors create cost, it was therefore decided to limit the number of doctors. The unintended result was our present doctor shortage.

In order to cope with the shortage—which was especially acute in rural areas—foreign medical graduates were encouraged to come to Australia. Now about 40% of Australian doctors are foreign graduates. This helped the rural shortage, but the way the policy was implemented also created a time-bomb. The rural foreign graduates were required to serve about 10 years in the country before being granted general registration. This time limit is now coming to an end and so we can expect a mass migration of country doctors to the large cities. This will again leave the country areas short of doctors and produce a glut of doctors in the cities.

Another way the number of doctors was increased was by increasing the number of undergraduates being trained by our universities. This has produced two further problems:

- there are not enough postgraduate training positions to train the number of graduates and

- when these graduates are trained, there will not be jobs for all of them.

> *"when everyone is somebody, then no-one's anybody"*
> Gilbert & Sullivan, The Gondoliers

To understand why some politicians divert public funds from worthwhile objectives, we need to consider the educational upbringing of many of them.

Marx

> *"Have you read Marx?"*
> *"I'll give you red marks!"*
> from "Take it from Here" by Frank Muir & Denis Nordern

Labor Party members develop in an environment

steeped in the teachings of Karl Marx. Marx developed the theory of a class struggle, in which workers and capitalists were class enemies. He postulated that the workers would eventually subdue the capitalists and the world would live in harmony.

According to Marx, all capital (or wealth) is derived from the output of labor. The fruits of a worker's labor were appropriated from him and added to the capitalist's store of wealth. In Marx's words, capital is "crystallized labor in the abstract".

Now Marx did recognize that factors of production such as a lathe or loom did multiply a laborer's productive output but, as capital was only crystallized *labor*, he never considered that the supplier of the lathe or loom had any right to reward for that supply.

The Jesuits have a saying: "Give me the child until the age of seven and I will give you the man". The same principle applies to the unionist steeped in socialist tradition. As one with some experience in the field, I can assure you that it is very difficult to divorce one's self from the fears and noble aspirations that have been drilled into one as a child. Many union executives see employers as thieves and exploiters of vulnerable workers.

Councils

I was once a councillor on a city council. At the time, the council officers had a penchant for creating traffic roundabouts. These roundabouts were often in rather strange geographical locations—but that's another story. What interested me was the cost. Each roundabout was priced at between $80,000 and $100,000. Frankly I could not see how a stone circle could cost so much, and nobody could ever satisfy me that it did. Well, in order to build each roundabout, tenders were sought. When tenders closed, the council officers would allot the work to selected companies. These companies were not always the cheapest. When I asked why, I was told that the companies were chosen because they did good work. One has to ask: why bother asking for tenders when you have already decided who is going to get the job?

Another item of interest to me when I was on council was the inability to extract information from council officers. At one stage I asked how many employees the council had, what they did and what they were paid. "Sorry, I can't give you that information", the officers said. "The unions wouldn't allow it." So I wrote to the State Minister of Local Government in the then Labor government to ask for his support in getting the information. His reply, in essence, was: "Yes, you are entitled to that information but I'm not going to make them give it to you".

The question arises as to why councilors, or anyone else for that matter, are not permitted to know how many people are employed by a council. One possibility that readily springs to mind is that the council is employing *ghost* workers, that is, workers who collect pay but do no work. Even an audit of council finances will not ensure that Mr. Michael Mouse does, in fact, provide any services to the council. Nor would the auditor know, or indeed care, whether Mr. Mouse used most of his pay to give generous donations to his preferred political party.

This same pattern can be seen in the recent and notorious "Building the Education Revolution" cock-up. Much money was allocated to building school halls and the like for schools—whether the schools needed them or not! This appeared like a good idea at the time, although it went a little awry. However, it can be seen as another form of mischievous funds diversion.

In New South Wales, the government decreed that work on public projects must be done by designated builders. It was later found that these builders charged up to twice the rate that private builders acting for private schools charged where proper tendering for projects was enforced.

Why weren't public schools allowed to get the contractors who offered the cheapest constructions? Why were certain firms favored? One is tempted to ask if some of this money found its way to less deserving projects. At local and state government levels we see a similar mystical disappearance of large amounts of public funds.

You might have noticed that the Labor Party is persisting with the drive to recognize local government in the constitution. This would enable the Federal government to directly fund them. Guess why? If you feel that an insufficient amount of your tax money is being hived off by political parties, you know how to vote!

We don't need councillors or local councils. Councilors mainly do what they are told by council officers. This is because very few of them have managerial or financial experience. As councilors are more attuned to social engineering than good management, the cost to the community of their social interference and mismanagement is enormous. Let the areas run by council officers fall under the purview of state governments without the interference (and cost) of posturing amateur politicians.

A similar diversion of funds has occurred with the Medicare reform (read "cock-up"). The health care system has become a milch cow for bureaucrats. When attempts are made to decrease the number of unnecessary employees, the cry invariably goes up that poor people are being put out of work. The fact that thousands of needy people are being deprived of their rightful treatment because of this inappropriate diversion of funds is never considered.

3 | THE ECONOMY

There are three areas of our economy that might seem unrelated to health care. However, an understanding of these areas is very important if we want to minimize cost and increase efficiency of our social security. These areas are *taxation, medical negligence* and *superannuation*.

Taxation

The financial picture of the average household can be likened to a golden river passing in front of its door. The stream coming down consists of income in the form of salary, interest, dividends and so forth. The stream passing by consists of money that one is obliged to pay out in the form of tax, rent and living expenses. Thus a citizen has access to merely a bucket of money from the passing stream. To some people this is a small or fixed amount.

But there are some (such as banks and doctors) who have the ability to increase the quantity that ends up in their bucket as circumstances dictate. If, for example, a tax is increased, the lucky ones can maintain (or even increase) their income by increasing their fees.

Governments often increase taxation rates and assume that the revenue derived will be proportional to the increase. But the result is usually much less revenue than calculated because taxpayers inevitably take action to avoid or decrease the effect of the impost (the Newton effect noted earlier).

Another interesting, but little understood, quirk of taxation is that there is no guarantee that the person on whom the tax is levied is the person who ends up paying the tax. For example, many years ago the state governments introduced a *Financial Institutions Duty* (FID) and the federal government introduced the *Bank Accounts Debit Tax* (BAD). These were taxes designed to affect only the banks. But what did the banks do? They simply passed the tax on to customers. Even worse for government, the banks highlighted the government tax at the bottom of every customer's bank statement. So, not only did the governments fail to get money from the banks as planned; they were punished for trying. This was because every customer could see that the government was raiding their savings and taxing them on money they had already paid tax on. FID and BAD thus sank silently beneath the waves of time. Today, when banks are making enormous profits, people are again clamouring to tax the banks further. We are likely to see the same pass-on manoeuver if the government is stupid enough to repeat the same routine.

There are contractors who are aware of this manoeuver and use it to their own advantage. They offer to do a job more cheaply if the customer does not want a receipt. One doesn't have to be a Rhodes Scholar to realize that this is outrageous tax avoidance. Hence all honest citizens insist on being given a receipt to ensure that those they contract contribute their fair share to the treasury.

But wait a minute! If you insist on a receipt you will end up paying more. This might ensure that the contractor pays the correct tax. But guess who is really paying the tax? You.

No greater love hath any man than he who would pay the tax of his neighbor.

When advocating that some section of the community should have their taxes increased, it is wise to consider whether this will have the slightest effect on the entity being taxed. There are some entities that cannot pass on tax increases to others (apart from the average luckless taxpayer). One such group is mining companies who make their profits from overseas buyers. Increases in taxes on profits derived from overseas buyers do not rebound on local citizens. But when attacking this little goldmine, one must consider what the mining companies might do to offset the attack. A close-down of mines with the loss of significant local jobs is one likely response.

Medical negligence

Negligence originally required that a person or entity:

- had a duty of care
- breached that duty and
- damage occurred as a result of that breach.

In medicine, the required standard of care is not clearly defined. In the past, the courts accepted that a medical act was not negligent if it followed a practice common amongst doctors. However, as many patients could only obtain compensation if negligence was proven, the courts have now taken the position that they would deem an act to be negligent if, in the view of the court, it was negligent. This meant that a medical practice could now be deemed negligent even if every doctor in the country practiced in that way. Thus the range of malpractice litigation has been extended.

Medical malpractice insurance is an area of significant cost to the health system. On the surface, it would seem that doctors are the ones shouldering the burden of compensation for medical mishaps. What is not realized is that the government is supporting a major insurance and legal industry as part of its health payments. *This is not immediately obvious because the money goes from government to these industries indirectly.*

The circus works as follows: doctors pay insurance premiums to support a large insurance industry. The insurance industry passes this money (after deductions for profit, salary and running expenses) on to the legal fraternity and to injured patients. But the government ultimately pays all of this because (a) doctors set their fees to cover the premiums and (b) the government pays the doctors for their services.

Medical malpractice insurance was originally created by doctors. Doctors see the results of medical damage first hand and don't always like the results. A mechanism to protect patients against damage was therefore instituted. This has now become compulsory, but the cost is wasteful. It can be as much as $100,000 a year for some doctors (for example, neurosurgeons).

Courts award damages for medical negligence on the assumption that the victim would need money to pay for on-going medical treatment as well as to sustain themself. But the government continues to pay for medical treatment *irrespective of whether the cost of treatment was included in the payout.* Thus any compensation award not only stuffs the coffers of the legal fraternity. It also amounts to a lottery win for the patient.

Doctors' fees could be significantly reduced if they didn't have to cover malpractice insurance.

"No fault" legislation

If a principle of "medical damage" were introduced into legislation, the superfluous costs to government mentioned above could be removed. Such a principle puts patient need before proof of negligence. Indeed, it does away with the notion of negligence in assessing damages.

Patients are often damaged by medical procedures without there being any negligence on the part of the doctor. However, at present the patient can only obtain compensation if they can prove negligence in a court of law. They may have to wait years to get into court only to find that negligence is not proven and they end up with nothing.

A damaged person needs immediate help, whether they are hit by a car or dive into the sea and break their neck. As soon as a patient is medically injured, a specialist doctor should assess the extent of the injury and stipulate the needs of the patient. Financial help should then be provided by the government within days.

Moving the focus from negligence to patient need carries a further benefit. In the case of medical interventions, doctors would no longer be inclined to wrongly minimize the severity of the assessed damage (as they might do in order to avoid an increase in their own malpractice liability). If there is any criminality in the cause of the injury, the matter can be referred to the courts at a later time.

Defensive medicine

An unintended consequence of medical malpractice insurance and litigation is a practice known as *defensive medicine*. If a doctor is likely to be sued for making a mistake or missing a diagnosis, they will take extra measures to avoid these errors. This, of course, is laudable—but do the costs outweigh the benefits?

For example, a person who presents with a stomach ache may be given numerous blood tests and even X-rays or a gastroscopy rather than a simple antacid. One would hate to miss a stomach cancer, but such a patient will inevitably return if the antacid doesn't work. All these unnecessary tests add to the cost of health care and, if the practice is unchecked, may eventually cripple the economy. Moreover, there is no guarantee that a battery of tests will always lead to a correct diagnosis. If doctors were left to practice medicine rationally, some mistakes would be made. That is inevitable. But there would be a significant reduction in the cost of health care.

The government is always complaining of doctors over-servicing patients. Well, if the government removed the legal threats to rational medical practice, doctors would not feel pressured to over-service.

Superannuation

Superannuation may not seem to be in any way related to health care, but it is—*indirectly*. In the 2013 Federal Government budget, nearly 35% of all government expenditure was earmarked for social security. Any decrease in the cost of social security—which can be brought about by improving superannuation coverage and thereby reducing the numbers dependent on Commonwealth assistance—must improve the economy. And a better economy permits more money to go to health care and decreases the numbers depending on Commonwealth assistance.

Why do we all want to accumulate money and

other assets? We live in an adversarial society—we need to look to own interests as nobody else will do it for us. Thus we all try to accumulate assets to protect ourselves against poverty in old age. But the purpose of superannuation is to enable us to do just that.

Many people hoard assets well beyond their needs. They accumulate numerous properties and share portfolios and, in doing so, sequester money from general circulation. If this money were freed, there would be more finance available for socially valuable uses (such as building necessary infrastructure). But in order to free this finance, those hoarding assets must be guaranteed the protection and security that their assets presently provide.

If people were guaranteed a comfortable retirement, there would be no need to accumulate property at the expense of younger people who have a justifiable need for property. Property would become more available and hence more affordable. Nor would there be any need to accumulate shares in public companies. The present gambling house that is the stock exchange would then be used less in the wasteful pursuit of paper wealth and more in the productive expansion of industry and the subsequent creation of employment.

The initial idea of private superannuation was sound. But because the government failed to consider the consequences of its legislation, the system has been abused and it has failed to meet its sensible objectives. For example, at the age of 65 a person with private superannuation can withdraw all their funds, spend the lot on what they please and then apply for government support. Further, anyone over 65 can pay up to $35,000 of earnings into superannuation, pay tax on it of 15% instead of the usual 45%, and then immediately withdraw the remainder (which they can spend as they please). So the existence of superannuation does not mean that it will necessarily be used for the purpose for which it was created.

Private superannuation funds can also be embezzled by fast-talking investment salesmen or by anyone else who can get their hands on the money. It can also be lost if it is used to play the stock market and the stock market takes a dive.

There is also enormous wastage of superannuation funds due to the overheads of superannuation funds and also due to the funds creaming off large amounts as management fees.

All governments would prefer citizens to pay the maximum tax that can be extracted and, from then on, look after themselves. We thus see politicians finding ever new and ingenious ways to raid private superannuation funds. Unfortunately, pretty well every dollar that politicians extract from superannuation funds becomes a dollar that the government has to pay out to support the superannuant later on. But that is a problem for a future government, not for this one.

Thus encouraging private superannuation does not necessarily reduce the government's liability to look after retirees in the future. Government control of superannuation would eliminate the possibility of diversion of superannuation funds to fund managers, investment salesmen or stock market collapses. In this way, retirement finance could be guaranteed and government would have more finance available to develop the country.

4 | HOSPITALS

Prior to the introduction of Medibank—later renamed *Medicare*—the medical profession had resisted attempts to nationalize health services. Because of this opposition, government authorities began removing doctors from positions of influence in the hospital system. This was a nationwide phenomenon. Today we have no advisors in hospitals who know what is required for safe and efficient patient care.

Needless to say, relations between doctors and government became a tad strained. The administrative antagonism toward doctors did not cease even with the introduction of Medibank. Some doctors who had worked in the same hospital for many years were re-interviewed in order to justify their continuing appointment. The purpose of such interviews was purely intimidatory.

A major feature of the *Medibank Act* was that it broke the traditional doctor–patient relationship. Doctors would no longer have a direct relationship with public patients. This was done by legislating two contracts:

1. *A contract between the patient and the public hospital*

Hospitals, by law, had to accept any patient who chose to be a public patient—even if they were privately insured. Moreover, the doctor could not bill the patient for services.

2. *A contract between the hospital and the doctor*

A patient who chose to be treated as a public patient no longer had the right to be treated by the doctor of their choice. Instead they would be treated by a doctor designated by the hospital (or a person delegated by that doctor).

Another way that doctors were removed from positions of authority and oversight was by replacing the Medical Superintendent with a politically appointed manager. Originally, the most senior officer in any hospital was the Medical Superintendent. But this seniority was more fragile than anyone suspected at the time. One day, a hospital manager who happened to have both medical and accounting qualifications decided that he would take over from the Medical Superintendent. The method was devilishly simple. All he did was order that the hospital stationery should now place his name in a position senior to that of the Medical Superintendent. From then on, he was the senior officer! Thus Medical Superintendents were rapidly sidelined and replaced by hospital managers. This meant that control of hospital policy now shifted from medical needs to the financial objectives of government.

Unfortunately, the flip side of sidelining doctors was that doctors were no longer available to give expert advice, and it wasn't long before administrators realized that they were facing big problems. They had no idea of medical priorities and the efficient deployment of finance to meet those needs. This was not helped by the financial limitations imposed by the government.

State governments soon realized that Medibank was becoming very expensive and they began to decrease funding to hospitals. (Personally, I thought this was a good idea at the time because there was much wastage in the hospital system and some pressure for efficiency was in order.) The governments noticed that the decrease in funding seemed to have very little effect on the delivery of health care. They therefore repeated the exercise time and time again. But there was a limit to how far you could reduce hospital funding. Obviously, there would come a time when a hospital would be so crippled that it would be unable to function.

Here is a story I was told it on good authority. There once was a small suburban public hospital in the electorate of one of our more illustrious prime ministers. One day, a health system bureaucrat observed that this hospital was making a profit. To a government bureaucrat, an unsaleable public asset that makes a profit is anathema. Detailed investigations revealed that the profits were generated because the manager had been accepting paying private patients in order to balance the books. Such behavior was not to be tolerated. Once the manager had been apprised of his public duty, he increased the ratio of public patients and restored the financial position of the hospital back into the red in line with other self-respecting public hospitals. So diligent were his efforts that the bureaucrats ultimately had no choice but to close the hospital. Better no hospital than a renegade one!

One day a hospital manager approached a health minister and said: "I can't run the hospital on the money you give me". To which the minister replied: "Well if you can't, I'll find someone who can". Hospital managers, who apparently have less intestinal fortitude than Oliver Twist, soon learned not to ask for more. One manager did bite the bullet and spent the money required for his hospital to provide adequate and safe services. He didn't last long.

So now we had a situation where hospital managers had a choice: either work within the budget or lose your job! Unsurprisingly, almost every one of them chose the first alternative. Thus hospitals today always keep within their budgets. This might mean poor patient service, but what is more important: keeping your job or providing patient care? It was a no-brainer.

If you have a limited income and your costs go up, what do you do? You start by eliminating your greatest costs, don't you? Hospital managers are nothing if not managers and were right up to the mark on this one. A high-cost area in a public hospital is the operating theatre. So managers extended from one to four weeks the period operating theatres are closed over Christmas. That, of course, saved money. But guess what it did to surgical waiting lists? At about March, the managers revisited their anticipated budgets and again noted that a blow-out was on the horizon. So they repeated their original success and closed the theatres for one or two weeks in June. And surprise, surprise—the surgical waiting lists went up yet again.

Most public hospitals now have beds and even wards closed.

With the removal of doctors from administrative positions in hospitals, it was now open slather for administrators to use hospital finances as they saw fit. In order to save money, operating theatre staff may be lucky to get milk, dry biscuits and coffee powder. However, they occasionally do get special treats. Sometimes profuse trays of three-tiered gourmet sandwiches appear. These are the left-overs from managerial conferences held the previous night. You can't expect management to work on an empty stomach!

As the overriding brief of administrators is to stay within budget, they no longer need to seriously consider the medical needs of patients or doctors. If a doctor needs new equipment, an administrator can say that the hospital is over-budget and so cannot afford it. A blind eye can be turned to the fact that patients might now have to wait for years for pain-relieving operations. And by delaying surgery to ill patients, their health becomes even more critical, with the result that the cost of their surgery and subsequent care also increases.

The lack of medical oversight of hospital operations also guarantees that any diversion of funds will never be questioned. Indeed, if one examines the annual reports of most public hospitals, there is no way of determining if moneys have been properly spent or found their way into extraneous pockets.

But waiting lists came back to bite politicians on the bum. Reducing the waiting lists became the political mantra of the day. The first ploy was to redefine a waiting list. If a patient was given a definite time for their operation—let's say 12th October 2024—they were technically no longer on a waiting list. They might be waiting—and waiting for a long time—*but they were not on the waiting list*. But the issue would not go away. Something had to be done. Reducing waiting lists had to be funded in some way, so doctors were paid premium rates to increase their surgical output. As a result, the money saved by ward closures during holiday periods was soon more than overtaken by the increased cost of reducing waiting lists.

And the circus goes on: theatres close, waiting lists expand, doctors get paid a premium to reduce the lists, budgets are threatened, theatres close, waiting lists expand and so on ad infinitum. But I'm a doctor, so don't think I am ungrateful. Unfortunately, I also see the effects on patients at first hand. Let me tell you that "a thousand hip replacements" on a sheet of statistics means nothing compared to one patient sitting across your desk with pain engraved on their face asking for an explanation as to why they have to wait two years for so-called *free* medical treatment.

It is to the advantage of all political parties to do

nothing about improving the health system. In this way, the opposition can always complain about the state of the system and its deficiencies and promise to improve them. The government, of course, does nothing. When the opposition becomes government, it also does nothing leaving the new opposition to complain. In this way, both parties can promise something at a forthcoming election without ever having to deliver.

In days of old, each public hospital had its own local administrative board, but the buck stopped with the Health Minister. This meant that there was a definite person who ultimately took responsibility and to whom one could take complaints. This, of course, created irritation for the minister and also exposed their inadequacies. Then someone got the bright idea of creating *regional health areas*. This had a two-fold benefit: it devolved responsibility to regional managers and it created the impression that advantages were being taken of efficiencies of scale. Although you can still approach the minister if you have a complaint—as in days of yore—your success is almost certainly thwarted. It works as follows:

- When you complain to the minister, they will tell you that they only deal with policy and that you should instead raise your complaint with the hospital manager.

- The hospital manager will tell you that this problem is not within their area of jurisdiction and that you should see the nursing manager.

- The nursing manager will refer you to a nurse in charge of a ward who will refer you on to someone else.

- Ultimately, you will need to consult the tea lady—only to find that she has recently been sacked as a financial efficiency move.

In other words, there is no one who will take responsibility for anything or, if there is, you will never get to them.

Hospital managers essentially have to lie to everyone. They have to lie to the Health Minister to save their jobs, and they have to lie to the broader public about the state of hospitals. "Why are there wards closed in your hospital?" you might ask. Answer: "Because we can't get nursing staff". *Lie*. There are hundreds of nurses available and unable to get work. But the hospitals do not advertise any positions because they do not have the funds to pay for them. If the managers asked for more funds, they would be sacked for not working within their budget.

As there is now no medical oversight of spending in hospitals, administrators can give jobs to people who aren't really needed. Hence when a government trumpets its increased spending on health care, what it is really doing is transferring more taxpayers' money into the pockets of its chosen bureaucrats. No increase in the funding actually finds its way to patient care.

So administrators came to take over positions of authority from doctors, but they had no basic plan to work from and no idea of the priorities required. This left them in a vulnerable position in respect to damages claims. In order to protect themselves, administrators devised and documented extensive protocols. Thus if a patient comes to grief, it could always be argued that everything was done by the book and hence the death was nobody's fault. Thus nurses and doctors spend much valuable time filling in unnecessary paperwork simply to protect the administration, time that could be better spent caring for the needs of patients. It has become more important to fill out a nursing care plan than to empty a patient's bed-pan.

Hospital managers also needed numerous personnel to devise the necessary protocols and to police them. Thus we gained thousands of unnecessary bureaucrats who do nothing more than interfere with the running of the health system. But not only do they interfere with health delivery, they also divert millions of dollars away from actual patient care.

Doctors, nurses and administrators tend to paper over the problems of the health system in order to minimize adverse effects. This usually means working longer and more dangerous hours, or using less ideal, but cheaper, treatments for patients. This situation is far from ideal.

Credentials committees

Up until the 1960s, any qualified doctor of good repute working in the catchment area of a Victorian public hospital had the right to admit patients to that hospital. Further, staff appointments to hospitals were decided by individual hospital boards.

In the early 1970s the Victorian government felt that this system produced a "closed shop" whereby excellent outside candidates were denied appointment in favor of the hospital favorites. The government introduced legislation to ensure that staff appointments were widely advertised and the best candidates appointed.

However, in order to protect their closed-shop control of positions, local doctors set up hospital accreditation committees. Such committees could deny an outsider with excellent qualifications an appointment by finding some flaw in their credentials. This also allowed those doctors already appointed to the hospital to protect themselves by stating that no further doctors were required. The credentials committees therefore established a restrictive trade practice under the guise of protecting medical standards. This is akin to Coles or Woolworths saying that no other supermarket should be allowed in a certain area because the main players are providing an adequate service. If Coles or Woolworths used this argument to prevent competition, they would surely be prosecuted.

Credentials committees thus successfully stonewalled the government's objectives and protected the financial monopoly of doctors already appointed. There is no reason why such credentials committees should continue to exist. *Indeed, there is no valid reason why any doctor of good repute with the appropriate qualifications should not be able to practice in any hospital at any time.*

By opening all hospitals to all qualified personnel, medical standards must increase. Personnel of poor standard would not attract enough work and hence be weeded out. At present doctors of poor standard can continue working in a hospital because no one is game to challenge their performance for fear of legal reprisal. With open competition, no doctor could take court action on the grounds that they were not referred enough work.

5 DOCTORS AND NURSES

In ancient Egypt, the healing arts were the province of the priestly class. As time went by, the medical and theological divisions separated so that priests tended to the soul while doctors tended the body. Even today doctors are accorded a prestige somewhere between God and man. Indeed, many patients are afraid to offend their doctor in case the doctor may not tend them when their life is in the balance. Even politicians are reticent to contradict doctors for fear of divine retribution. This allows the profession a fair degree of latitude when it comes to bluff, helped along by the fact that doctors have maintained a degree of secrecy about the mysteries of medicine.

About 50 years ago, 3–5% of students reached university level. The kind-hearted government decided that it would be a good thing if everybody reached that academic level. But, again, nobody thought of the consequences.

> *"when everyone is somebody, then no-one's anybody"*
> Gilbert & Sullivan, The Gondoliers

In medicine and nursing, we are now producing too many graduates. Already, nurses who have spent three years training find that they cannot get employment. The lag in medicine is slower but the proverbial excreta is about to hit the fan. Although there is, apparently, a deficit of about 30,000 general practitioners, this deficit will quickly disappear, for the medical schools are beginning to churn out graduates at a prodigious rate. But they are churning out more than is necessary. There will be no postgraduate training positions for many of these new graduates.

Further, a great number of foreign medical graduates have been imported. These graduates are indentured to work in rural areas for 10 years before they can attain general registration (which allows them to practice anywhere). Many of these foreign graduates are coming to the end of their indenture. The expectation is that many of them will seek work in the major cities.

The obvious conclusion is that we are facing a glut of doctors. And what will be the natural consequence of that? Doctor's fees will skyrocket to ensure that each doctor can make a decent living. If you think medicine is expensive now, just wait a few years.

In the 1960s, a surgeon could become qualified four years after graduating. Today, it can take ten to fifteen years. How has this inordinate extension of training occurred? To answer this question, we need to understand the history of our health system and the response of the specialist medical colleges.

There have always been specialist medical colleges—such as the College of Surgeons and the College of Physicians—but these were essentially elite old-boys clubs. Entrance into a specialist college was by examination or, exceptionally, by election. The examinations were designed to establish some degree of quality, but they were also designed to ensure that those already in the specialty had some control over who entered their august establishment.

Up until the early 1960s, any graduating doctor was legally entitled to perform any medical procedure they wanted to without needing to be certified by any specialist college. By the mid-1960s, the number of undergraduates had increased significantly, which subsequently caused many graduates to gravitate towards the specialties. But with more specialists, the workload per specialist would decrease, and hence it was feared that the viability of each specialist practice could become marginalized.

Colleges

Surgery has traditionally been the glamor specialty of medicine, and so the first college to feel the pain of this increase in graduates seeking a specialist niche was the College of Surgeons. The College took a number of steps to limit the number of trainees. Many of these steps did limit the numbers in the short term, but at a significant social and economic cost. Moreover, those steps were more of a delaying tactic than an effective method of reducing graduates, for the same number eventually graduated, but at a later time.

The argument of the College, however, was quite reasonable: If there are too many surgeons there will not be enough work for each and the eventual financial rewards will not be worth the effort. But as the College was acting in isolation from the general economy, it did not consider the ultimate effects of its strategies.

Teaching

All so-called teaching in Australia amounts to *lecturing*— and there is a difference!

- Teaching implies that knowledge is transferred from the teacher and implanted into the mind of the student.

- Lecturing implies that the lecturer simply places knowledge in front of the student. What the student does with that knowledge is a matter for them and their god.

The average teacher regards their work done once they have placed relevant knowledge before the class. But if a teacher is to teach efficiently, they must not only place knowledge before students: they must also check to see that the student understands it and has absorbed it. But student tests today are designed more as academic hurdles than as mechanisms to inform teachers of their own deficiencies. If teachers used tests to note the gaps exhibited by each student, and then filled in those gaps, their teaching would be much more efficient.

Medical teaching is even worse than general teaching. After an examination, a medical student never knows what they did right and what they did wrong. This is because they never have their paper returned. Nor does the examiner take the time to ensure that the student eventually comes to fully comprehend the material examined.

This system has allowed the medical profession to pick and choose who it will admit to its ranks and avoids the embarrassment of a candidate challenging an assessment if they fail. But such a system also lacks clear standards. It also explains why we are now seeing inadequate treatment and the appearance of rogue doctors. Further, it explains how we have created the present shortage of doctors. The government's reaction to the shortage has been to open more training positions and to admit more foreign graduates. But the colleges can simply offset this by extending training time.

Surgical training

Prior to the late 1950s, any person who had the secondary

school qualifications for entry to university could enrol as a medical student. As the numbers wishing to study medicine increased, a quota on the intake was introduced. At the time I graduated (1964), the training period for a surgeon was two postgraduate resident years and two years of specialized surgical training. In the 1960s, the Royal College of Surgeons in England deemed a two-year apprenticeship under a competent surgeon as adequate to acquire the requisite skills. But the aim of the colleges in Australia has been to delay the qualification of graduates by prolonging training time. This was a bottler. Just keep adding a year of training and surely a number of potential candidates would get the hint and pull out. There really is no limit to how far the training period could be extended— at least, that is, until someone gets the message and puts a stop to it.

Nowadays, medical graduates would be lucky to enter the surgical training program with less than four postgraduate resident years. They are then required to do four years of basic training plus a further two years of advanced training. However, if you itemize the skills required for any specialty and allot an adequate training time to acquire each one, you will clearly see that a training period exceeding 3 years for any specialty (including surgery) cannot be justified.

The present postgraduate courses are replete with unnecessary academic garbage. For example, in the college of anesthetists, candidates are required to submit a "formal project". This is essentially a research project. I am not against research, but why does a clinical anesthetist need to have research experience? Let those whose scientific bent is toward research train for and indulge their passion. Over the past decade, I don't know of one such project that has catapulted the science of medicine into the next century.

This is not to decry the efforts of my younger colleagues. It is simply to point out the wasteful stupidity of creating work for work's sake and the futility and cost of looking for answers to questions that no one would otherwise bother to ask.

Presently, our young doctors are having years of their lives unnecessarily wasted. The cost to the community of this unnecessary training time—and an artificial limiting of manpower—is enormous. We are importing large numbers of doctors from overseas. In order to practice as specialists, the overseas graduates have to enter the same examination system that excludes so many locals. Many foreign doctors also have visas that require them to return to their country of origin if they do not pass the local exams within a specified period. The disruption to their lives in coming to this country and then being failed because of an iniquitous examination system is simply unfair. The bad name that Australia is getting for this gross abuse of skilled personnel will certainly cost us dearly in the future.

Accredited training positions

In order to limit the number of training positions, the various colleges designated certain hospitals as accredited for training purposes. Some such hospitals were accredited for the entire training course of a specialist; others had limited accreditation.

To train a specialist, there are three requirements:

1. a candidate
2. a trainer and
3. adequate facilities to provide the training.

You do not need to have accredited hospitals to provide these needs. In fact, if the trainees could choose their places of training, there would be more rural trainees (as rural consultants are more interested in retaining trained staff than city consultants).

We also have the absurdity of "non-accredited" training positions. This implies that a candidate is being trained but not trained at the same time. These positions were only devised in order to provide lackeys for consultants without the danger of having too many candidates graduate.

Cost of training

Increasing the cost of training seemed to be a winner.

In 2011, the Australasian College of Surgeons had 1,224 trainees on its program. The income to the college from training and examination fees was $17.8 million. This amounts to an average annual cost of over $14,000 to each trainee. Now this average figure might include all sorts of extra odds and sods, but it does give one a ballpark figure of how much the College extracts from its trainees.

In 2013 the fee to sit the College of Surgeon's exam is $6,850. No doubt the college can justify this fee—but couldn't it be cheaper? There is no reason why candidates need to attend a specific examination center, nor is there any reason why candidates cannot be tested on practical knowledge during their training. In fact, there is no reason why the examinations under the present conditions need to be held at all.

The expense of this training is ultimately met by the government. There is also the cost to the taxpayer of two doctors doing the one job when the consultant is required to also be present while a competent trainee does a procedure. And since each trainee surgeon is doing this for 5 to 10 years more than they need to, the cost to the trainee and to society is enormous.

Exams

An advantage that all medical colleges have is that they never provide a clear syllabus. Thus a candidate can never be sure of what they are required to know and so can easily be failed on the whim or design of an examiner. At one stage, the pass rate for the first-part surgery exam was as low as 15%.

There is no documentary proof that a candidate has, in fact, failed. Because of the secrecy of the examination system, no candidate can challenge their results. Marked papers are not returned to candidates for them to see where they went wrong. They cannot go to an impartial umpire to argue for fair treatment. There are no documents to take and no record of any harassment they may have been subject to. For a price, a candidate is able to get a written report on their exam, but it is obviously absurd to pay for the same advice that you had already received for free. In fact, there is no guarantee that any examiner even looked at an exam paper. But then, if you want to keep your club exclusive, that's the way to do it.

Candidates for specialist postgraduate qualifications will certainly have an intelligence within the top 5% of the human race. So how is it that up to 50% have been known to fail a postgraduate exam at their first attempt? Would you send your child to a school that had an examination failure rate of 50%? Would you regard that school as one that was dedicated to the maintenance of high standards?

There are three possible causes for such a failure rate:

1. *The candidate is unintelligent or uninterested.*

We have already dealt with the intelligence issue, so this is unlikely to be a factor. Further, the fact that the application fees for exams are exorbitant should deter the uninterested.

2. *The training is substandard.*

This is an understatement. There is no coherent structured training program in most of the specialties. Clinical tutors have no direction as to what needs to be taught and no advice on how to ensure that important material is inculcated. The trainees have log books, but these are not used to ensure that they have a comprehensive understanding of vital procedures. Trainees merely note that they have done a particular procedure without any indication as to whether they did it well or completely cocked it up. In fact, as long as the trainee took some part in the procedure, they can note it in their log book.

No trainee would dare complain about the methods being employed by the colleges because they would then find there are no training positions available to them. Where do they go then?

3. *The examination system is unfair.*

The unfair examination system is already exacting a human cost. One lady registrar returned from her second or third failed attempt to pass the anesthetic primary exam. She said to me at the time: "David, I don't know how many more relationships I can afford to throw away while I attempt to pass this exam". I never found out how many more she did throw away before she committed suicide.

When I have questioned the fairness of the examination system, the college seniors invariably asked me: "Don't you trust the examiners?" This answer is really a red herring because the examiners are only servants of a pre-determined process. They cannot make allowances for the fact that a candidate is nervous or confused as a result of the pressure of an examination. If the candidate doesn't answer enough questions correctly, they fail. It is not a matter of deciding what a candidate actually knows; it is more often a matter of ferreting out how much they don't know in order to fail them.

Another of my registrars was asked by an examiner how many methods he knew for determining the humidity in an operating theatre. (As an aside, I don't think I have seen more than two wet-bulb thermometers in theatres in almost 50 years of practice—and I have certainly never had occasion to use one). He said he knew of two. The examiner asked him to describe one of the methods. He began his explanation but before he had finished two sentences the examiner interrupted him and said: "No not that method, the other one". Can anyone really claim that the examiner had not already determined to fail him?

Such stories undermine trust in examiners. They accentuate the belief that the only reason for keeping exam results secret is to prevent others knowing that you have done something underhanded. If the exams are fair, why can't the candidates see that for themselves?

Standards

A standard, by definition, is something which is objective and against which one can compare like things. On this definition, it is hard to show that there really are any defined standards in medicine. The present system allows sub-standard candidates to be passed and good candidates to be failed. (I am not insinuating that this has been widespread throughout history of medicine, although that is a possibility.) It allows the specialist colleges to arbitrarily limit the numbers of doctors that are admitted to that specialty.

What we need is a system whereby the student rather than the teacher is the one of paramount importance, where the required knowledge is clear and the student is drilled until they know the information thoroughly and is confident in that knowledge. Where a consultant does not bring their trainee up to the required standard in the allotted time, it is the consultant—not the trainee— who should be sacked.

With air pilots, practical and theoretical training is given by instructors on an hourly fee basis. There is a clear syllabus, and theory exams—usually made up of multiple-choice questions—can be taken over the Internet. The results are returned to the candidate within minutes and it is clear which questions they got right and which they got wrong. A student pilot is required to get 80% on the initial theory test. If a question is answered wrongly, the student pilot is later required to satisfy an instructor that they now understand the correct answer. Hence, the student pilot must ultimately pass 100% of the theory test. Why can't doctors be examined in a similar way?

So how do you know if your doctor's knowledge is up to date? Well, frankly, you don't. But don't feel bad about that—for even doctors can't really tell. The latest medical posturing is called "Continuing Professional Development" (CPD). This is a system whereby doctors attend lectures, seminars and training sessions for which they are awarded points. These points are known lovingly in the profession as "brownie points"—mainly because they are a childish waste of time and have nothing to do with ensuring quality of medical care. But they do avoid re-certification.

There are two major disadvantages to the re-certification to senior specialists:

1. Young doctors have minds like steel traps and would pass any reasonable test in a heartbeat. This would allow too many newcomers into the specialties too quickly. It would decrease the power of the colleges to maintain the artificial scarcity which limits competition.

2. The leaders themselves would have to be re-tested regularly. If you want to see a senior doctor perform a sudden involuntary explosive bowel movement, simply tell him that they will be required to re-sit their specialist exams within 6 months or lose their registration. The reality is that virtually no specialist could pass the exams that their successors are required to sit in order to gain admission to the specialty. Re-certification strikes terror into the hearts of all doctors. This is because the exams are not based on any clear idea of what knowledge is required and anyone who has passed through the adversarial process of gaining specialist certification has no wish to flagellate themselves yet again.

However, if standards were clearly defined and all efforts were directed to ensuring that everyone was brought up to those standards, there would be no fear of any re-certification process. In this way, we could be sure that all doctors were proficient at all times. What is more, all doctors would know—and be proud of the fact—that they were maintaining the highest of standards.

Schedule fee

By 1970, pressure was mounting on governments to assist patients with the cost of medical care. The Gorton government introduced the concept of the "common fee". This meant that the government would pay a rebate to the patient of about 85% of the fee for a given medical service if that fee was the fee commonly charged by doctors for that service.

Two specialties stood out in respect to common fees:

- Ear, nose and throat surgeons were clever enough

to raise their common fees substantially prior to the introduction of the new measure.

- Obstetricians, on the other hand, did not. This meant that obstetricians were rebated the same amount for looking after a woman during her pregnancy and delivery as an ENT surgeon got for placing grommets in the ears of three or four children. Thus there was an unfair disparity of fees between varying specialties.

With the advent of Medibank, the common fees were listed and costed by government, and each became known as the *schedule fee*.

As time went by and inflation rose, doctors began requesting an increase in the schedule fees. Naturally, the government was not keen to have inordinate increases and felt that an independent fees tribunal should be set up. This worked well for a short time, but it soon became apparent that the cost to government was rising faster than the government wanted. The independent tribunal was thus abolished.

Since that time, the schedule fee has increased at only about half the rate of increase in general wages. This has led to doctors increasing their fees independently of the government schedule, so that privately insured patients are now hit with an extra cost on top of their insurance. Originally, the government legislated to prevent doctors colluding to set higher fees. Thus, anti-collusion (anti-union) legislation was introduced against doctors (but not against unions). But the Australian Medical Association (AMA) easily bypassed this legislation by stepping in and recommending the fees that doctors should charge for their services. As these recommended fees could be justified on a commercial basis, they could not easily be challenged.

The rebatable fee structure for doctors needs to be re-evaluated to ensure that all doctors maintain reasonable incomes no matter what specialty they choose to enter.

Nurses

A reason why nurses can't get jobs these days is due to the egocentricity of senior members of the nursing profession. In order to increase the prestige of nursing, it was felt that nurses should have university degrees.

In 1970, I was an anesthetic resident in the USA. America had already introduced college education for nurses, and the hospitals were not happy with it. The hospitals were crying out for the superior *clinically trained* nurses from England and Australia.

But in Australia it would be different. Every proven overseas medical cock-up has been introduced here on the assumption that we would be different. The status of nurses was going to be exalted. The fact that nursing is a hands-on occupation rather than an academic one never seemed to occur to those who wished to increase their own status. Patients, for some unaccountable reason, prefer nurses who can nurse rather than those who can devise extensive nursing care plans.

At the time of the proposed transition from hospital training to university training of nurses, a sailor rang a talk-back radio station. He pointed out that sailors used to be trained at sea, over a period of three years. Then the navy decided to train them on-shore before going to sea. Thus they did some preliminary years training on-shore *but still needed three years at sea before they were competent*.

The proponents of university training for nurses would hear of no objections. Now we have nurses training for three years at university before graduating. Many then find that they don't like nursing after all. Previously, they found this out in their first year of hospital training. So now we have many wasted lives.

Also, because the universities admit as many nursing trainees as they wish, there is no quota of trainees.

Previously, the hospitals only had a limited number of training positions, so they could not train excessive numbers. Now we have an enormous percentage of university-trained nurses who can't find jobs.

Nursing administration

If one enters the office of a Nursing Unit Manager (NUM), one might notice a tall bookshelf against a wall. This contains, as one might expect, a number of books. But on the top shelf, there is usually a two-meter line of folders each about 5 centimeters thick. These folders contain important protocols, giving direction on pretty much everything. Now, there is nothing wrong with knowing what is expected, but two obvious questions spring to mind:

1.   Does anyone read these protocols?
2.   How much time and money has been taken out of the health budget to generate them?

Administrators obviously take the view that common sense is not all that common.

As a result of the newly devised protocols, nurses are diverted from nursing duties to devise nursing care plans which would arguably be unnecessary if they simply had time to look to the obvious needs of their patients. The diversion of finance from the coal face to the back room also leaves us with an inadequate number of trained nurses. So not only do we have fewer nurses, but those available spend less time nursing. This results in an overload of work on the nurses available and a danger to the patients.

For all the plans and protocols, there is no evidence that patient care has improved over the years. But there is evidence that more accidents are occurring in hospitals today than 30 years ago.

6 | CONCLUSION

What we have seen is the damage done to the Australian health system by the opportunism of politicians followed by the self-protective responses of the medical profession. There is much that must change if total chaos is to be avoided. The warring parties must recognize that the present system is economically unsustainable. There must be a reorganization to decrease wastage and inefficiency. There is an urgent need to assess the likely requirement of doctors for the future; otherwise we are heading for a medical and economic catastrophe—if we aren't there already!

> *For they have sown the wind and they shall reap the whirlwind*
>
> Hosea 8.7

It is said that the function of government is to perform those social necessities that would not otherwise be provided by the private sector. In the private sector, much of the administration is done free of charge (by the owner of a business). Also the owner is more aware of efficiency and of the need to keep costs low. These administrative and managerial functions are rarely done well, or at all, in the public sector. Hence, the more commercial and social activity that is performed by the private sector the more efficiently the country runs.

As far as the health care system is concerned, it is to the advantage of both opposing political parties to do nothing to improve it. The reason for this is that an opposition can always complain about the deficiencies of the system and promise to improve them. Meanwhile, the government does nothing. When the opposition becomes government, it also does nothing leaving the new opposition with ammunition to complain. This is a win–win situation for both parties: governments never have to do very much to correct the health system and oppositions always have a political argument for re-election.

The present Australian health system (Medicare) was introduced for naked political purposes. And since its primary purpose was to buy votes—rather than to provide an efficient and sustainable health system—it has gross deficiencies.

To provide rebates for trivial illnesses certainly buys the votes of a large number of citizens. But it diverts money from more worthy needs requiring major medical costs. For example, rebating patients for coughs and colds diverts money from the pool needed for knee or hip replacements.

Because *all* medical costs are rebated, patients can see their doctor for a medical certificate in order to have a day off work, or to ask for tests that aren't medically necessary but which make the patient feel healthy. Doctors are also unrestricted in the tests they can order. If one is ordering a full blood examination, one may as well have liver, kidney and blood-fat tests done at the same time. This inordinate wastage of money is crippling the Medicare system. If no incentive to contain costs is implemented, the system will collapse.

I suggest that the following three policies will avert the catastrophe:

1. There should be no rebate of medical costs, either by government or insurance companies, if the total cost is less than, say, $2000 in a year. In this way, patients would be deterred from seeking unnecessary medical attention. It would also limit the inordinate use of special tests by doctors. If a test was being considered and the patient knew that they would be paying for it, the patient would question the need for the test. It would also deter patients from asking for tests purely to see if there was something wrong with them.

2. Let patients be able to privately insure themselves or their families for the cost of medical expenses when those costs are between $2000 and $50,000 in any given year. Because of this limited liability on insurance companies, premiums could be cut drastically, thus making it affordable for patients to insure themselves.

Presently, government encourages private insurance as an underhand method to subsidize its own unsustainable system. It does this by requiring insurance companies to provide cover for every person and to insure them at the same cost. Clearly, some patients need more medical care than others and hence the healthy patients are subsidizing those who are more risky. This is called community rating.

If enough people leave private insurance, the government will be forced to remove the extortionate community rating and let insurance companies insure according to risk. That is, people will then be insuring themselves only and not every other medical cripple and his dog as well.

3. The government should cease subsidizing medical care except where patients cannot afford it or when annual medical expenses exceed $50,000 per year. This would immediately remove an enormous cost burden on government.

It cannot be emphasized enough that the only reason the government introduced universal "free" health care was to buy electoral votes. It never had anything to do with providing efficient affordable health care.

Regionalization of hospitals

As an efficiency measure, state governments bundled together groups of locally administered public hospitals under regional administrations. A similar approach was forced on local councils in order to decrease costs and increase efficiency. In itself, such amalgamation is admirable. However, with hospitals there is also a need to increase *functionality*. We presently have one such health administration stretching from the South Australian border to the eastern seaboard along the Murray River. Although providing some administrative efficiencies, this situation is not ideal.

The concept of regional administration is good, but it should be *functional* and not *geographic*.

We really need three tiers of hospital under the one administration:

1. *Local hospitals*

Such hospitals would provide first-aid local services in response to life-threatening emergencies (or example, heart attacks and major injuries). They could also deal with minor medical problems—such as coughs and colds—and perform minor operations.

2. *Regional hospitals*

These would treatment patients whose ailments are beyond the scope of the local hospitals. They would deal with major trauma and the longer-term treatment of severe medical conditions. They would have intensive care wards, sophisticated X-ray facilities and the ability to undertake major operations.

3. *Tertiary referral hospitals*

These would have facilities to cope with major medical problems as well as open-heart and neurological operations.

These three tiers need to be integrated so that patients who developed a need for the facilities of another level of hospital could be easily transferred from one to the other within their region. The hospitals need to be placed in areas of local need, not at distance from those who need them.

It would also require that doctors assigned to any hospital in the region could practice and operate at any of the other hospitals in that region. This would ensure that all patients and all doctors in the region would have access to the best facilities available. For example, a doctor working at a local hospital would not try to perform an operation at that hospital if the patient required the facilities of a regional hospital. The doctor would be able to transfer the patient to the regional hospital and operate on them there.

Hospital funding

There is a simple way to correct the hospital funding problem, but politicians would be unlikely to accept it as it would bring their hypocrisy into stark relief.

An *independent audit* of each hospital needs to be done according to the following guidelines:

1. What patients come to the hospital?
2. What services *is* this hospital providing?
3. What services *should* this hospital provide?
4. What services is this hospital providing that it should *not* be providing?
5. What personnel (doctors, nurses, administrators, and ancillary staff) are required to provide the services that the hospital should be providing?
6. What facilities (buildings, equipment) are required to service the needs of the hospital?

Estimate the cost of the above—*that is the funding required.*

If a minister refuses to provide the funds required, they must specify the elements that will not be funded so that the hospital managers can tell the press and the public: "These are what the community needs, and this is what the minister refuses to fund".

To simply deduct finance from a hospital to save money is stupidity. If you must pay $500 to register your car in order to use it on the road, it is nonsense to pay only $400 as a cost saving measure. Just as $400 does not allow you to drive your car on the road, underfunding a hospital does not allow it to work efficiently.

National database of medical professionals

We need to estimate what the populations of

various areas are likely to be in 10 years and how many general practitioners and specialists will be needed to service that need. We then need to set quotas on the number of local students to be trained and on the number of foreign graduates to be admitted.

An enormous drain on health system finances is the inordinate amount of unnecessary duplication and paperwork required by government and hospital authorities. Here are just two examples:

1. *Provider numbers*

Every doctor requires a separate provider number for each location at which they work. This means that every time a doctor begins work at a new site, they must apply to the government for a new provider number. Just think of the clerical time (and doctor's time) wasted as a result. And that all costs money.

2. *Hospital credentials*

To become accredited at a particular hospital, a doctor must supply to the hospital authorities certified copies of their qualifications, evidence of medical registration, evidence of continuing medical education, copies of their driver's license and passport, evidence of lack of criminality and a clearance to work with children. In spite of the fact that all doctors must maintain evidence of continuing medical education as a pre-requisite for registration, each hospital requires separate evidence of exactly the same information. This must be repeated at every hospital or medical care facility at which the doctor works.

Why can't these requirements be kept in a central database (maintained, perhaps, by the medical registration board) and updated annually? Any restrictions on a doctor's right to practice could also be recorded in this database. In this way, anyone requiring any information about a doctor could obtain it with a simple phone call.

Training of doctors

The concern of doctors is that if too many doctors are trained there will not be enough work for those already in the profession to maintain their skills. This can be corrected by determining the numbers of doctors required and training that number. Consideration will need to be given to the numbers starting the course and then dropping out, overseas graduates immigrating and different doctors having different specialist interests.

The proper way to train any specialist is to list the procedures and knowledge required and then drill each candidate until they are proficient. This is not presently done because any intelligent doctor would easily reach any standard set and thus become competition to those already in the specialty.

The present system wastes many years of the lives of young doctors. It also results in specialists who are not confident in their abilities. Because there are no clear standards, the standard expected in any particular place is that of any petty martinet who has achieved a position of authority. And there is no way of measuring the competence of any of these petty martinets either.

We need to understand that young people entering the study of medicine are very bright. Through their school years, they have had no difficulty in passing exams. When they study medicine, they again pass without much effort. Then, suddenly, they begin to fail postgraduate exams. Psychologically, their confidence is shattered. They now come to question whether they are competent (having never experienced incompetence before). Little do they know that their failure in postgraduate exams is a political stratagem to keep specialist numbers low. It has nothing to do with their competence. But this treatment of our postgraduate doctors is leading to lack of confidence, harmful self-introspection and fear for their future. We must stop this authoritarian bullying from the senior members of the medical profession. Students and junior doctors must be nurtured, protected and given rapid graded responsibility until their confidence and competence are established.

We now have at least one generation of doctors who are already damaged. Their rate of suicide and use of harmful drugs is alarmingly high. The cost to the community of this damage and wastage is incalculable.

Because postgraduate "training" is really a process of limiting competition in the specialty, trainees are often made to feel like fools. A consultant might ask a question that the trainee cannot answer. The consultant's response almost invariably is "You should know that!" When you think of it, this retort is nonsense. If the trainee should know it, surely it is up to the consultant to make sure that they do. Hence we have a new breed of junior consultants who are unsure of themselves and who don't know if they know all that they should.

We need to change the emphasis of training such that the trainee is in the box seat. That is, the trainee will be given a clear idea of the required knowledge (the syllabus) and the consultant will be responsible for instilling that knowledge. If a consultant does not bring their trainee up to the required standard in the allotted time, it is the consultant who is sacked, not the trainee.

The right of specialist colleges to be examining bodies must be removed. Put simply, they have a vested interest in failing candidates. And because the exam system of the colleges is designed to keep people out rather than to train them, no candidate has any idea what they are required to know. There is no clearly defined syllabus that a candidate can refer to. When candidates eventually do pass, they really do not know whether they are up to an acceptable standard.

Postgraduate training for specialists does not have to be done in specially accredited hospitals. It can be done anywhere there is a competent trainer and adequate facilities. A suggested training format is:

Basic

a)   Four years of undergraduate studies
b)   Two clinical years to become a city GP (that is, one with readily available back-up)

Advanced

c)   One extra clinical year to become a country GP
d)   Three extra clinical years to become a specialist of any discipline

A suggested training format for specialists is:

a)   Pre-reading of the procedure by the candidate
b)   Tutorial concerning the procedure with a specialist
c)   Demonstration of the procedure by a specialist
d)   Specialist assists the candidate
e)   Candidate performs a minimum number of the procedures by himself with specialist back-up
f)   Candidate is tested on the procedure by three specialists who attest to the candidate's competence

Examinations

Theoretical knowledge could be tested via the

Internet and done anywhere. This eliminates the need for the candidate to take time off work or pay for expensive travel and accommodation. It also eliminates the need for examiners to travel to oversee the performance. A candidate could apply to sit for their exam at any time and be allotted a time and supervisor for the test. This time could be within one week of application.

If the required knowledge is clear, the results of the test could be returned to the candidate within minutes. If their score exceeds, say, 80% they are awarded a pass with the proviso that, at a later stage, a competent supervisor certifies that they clearly know the material relating to the questions they did not answer correctly.

Practical and procedural competence can be assessed by examining each required procedure after the candidate has performed a set number of such procedures satisfactorily (as described above).

Thus everyone could be guaranteed that every doctor was competent. Presently nobody, including the candidate, has any such guarantee. It would also ensure that training was efficient and that trainees reached competent standards in the least possible time.

Standards

By definition, a standard is a concrete objective against which one can measure other things. If you accept that, then it is clear that there are no standards in medicine. There are no books of standards to refer to. This is probably why judges have decided to assess medical negligence themselves.

Because colleges design their courses and exams to exclude rather than to train, the result is that the training is random and poor. When the doctor eventually gets their qualification, they have no reason to be confident that they have achieved any acceptable standard.

Trainees cannot be expected to know what is important in their learning. They need guidance to ensure that they don't waste time learning useless information. However, the processes of the colleges ensure that the trainee's time is wasted in exactly this manner, with the result that important knowledge is often missed and irrelevant material clogs up the trainee's brain.

The emphasis of medical training needs to be shifted. Presently, consultants dominate the trainees and make it clear that kissing the professor's posterior is the highway to success. Trainees need to be able to choose their trainers and training institutions. In this way, the teachers that properly train trainees will get the clientele while those that do not will be sidelined.

We now come to two areas which are not strictly related to health care but which are areas of great cost to government. A decrease in costs and wastage in these areas and a re-deployment of finance would allow much better health care to be provided and would decrease the tax burden on everyone.

Medical malpractice insurance

By abolishing the cost to doctors of malpractice insurance, millions of dollars now paid to bureaucrats, lawyers and insurance companies for unnecessary work can be saved.

Where a victim is paid $1million, they can simply put that money in a bank, derive bank interest of $50,000 per year and still have $1million when they die. Of course, the payout could also be dissipated by the patient or by anyone who has access to the patient's finances (such as relatives, financial advisors or fraudsters). No matter how much a victim is paid, the government still has to provide the funds for their continuing health care.

We should legislate to create a concept of "no-fault medical damage". Then if a patient suffers damage as a result of a medical treatment, they would automatically be compensated without the need to prove how it was caused or by whom.

The advantages to the patient would be twofold:

1. The patient could be assessed fairly and quickly by a doctor without that doctor fearing an increase in their malpractice premiums.

2. The patient would get help immediately, and not have to wait 2 or more years until the case gets into court (as is often the case now).

There would be two further cost advantages:

1. Doctors would no longer have to incorporate indemnity costs into their fee structure and this would lead to a lowering of fees and thereby a lesser cost to government.

2. Without the fear of litigation hanging over their heads, doctors could practice medicine according to real medical needs rather than ordering tests, referrals and procedures purely to avoid litigation.

Government would not have any increased cost as it is already paying all of the costs—either directly or indirectly. Indeed, its costs would be decreased once it removed the insurance and legal monkeys from its back.

Superannuation

Federal government outlays for social security now amount to about 35% of the budget. On the surface, private superannuation might seem to decrease the liability government to care for the aged, but this is a delusion. What I am about to describe will seem a little left-wing, but it would be advantageous providing that governments are prevented from raiding the preserved funds.

The following scenario suggests one way to make superannuation efficient for both government and superannuants:

1. Determine what amount each person needs for a comfortable retirement at a particular time. *Comfortable* does not mean filthy rich, but it must include enough to cover such costs as housing, food, clothes and an agreeable life-style.

   Let us make the following assumptions about retirement in the year 2040 and accept that these assumptions have been estimated on an actuarial (that is, statistical) basis:
   - The retirement age is now 70.
   - At that age, life expectancy is 15 years (that is, until age 85).
   - A retirement nest egg of $1.5 million is required to ensure a comfortable life.

2. Let each person contribute to a government scheme, tax free, whatever amount they wished until the nest egg limit is reached. Sensible people would then contribute to their Superannuation in their high-earning years (between, say, 40 and 60) in order to minimize their tax burden. And since superannuation would not be compulsory, no contributions would need to be made in the poorly-earning and child rearing years up (until the age of 40 or so).

3. This superannuation money would then be *quarantined* into a government investment fund

whose purpose is to invest in infrastructure (roads, fast trains, hospitals, etc.) and commercial development (such as financing the development of new products). In other words, the government investment would be directed to increasing the social wealth of the country. It would also decrease the need for high taxes to pay interest on loans which are presently used to provide this infrastructure. It would thus abolish the need for toll roads to finance private road construction.

In order to prevent the superannuation fund from being used for political pork-barreling, a two-thirds majority of parliament should be required to approve infrastructure projects and commercial developments financed from the fund.

4. Such a government superannuation fund would provide an interest-free loan to the government and would guarantee a certain annuity to the superannuant when they retired. There would be no deductions from the superannuant's savings in the funds for management and other expenses.

Interest payments would no longer be made to superannuants, but this would be offset by decreased taxes and better social infrastructure.

5. On retirement, the superannuant would be paid a guaranteed annual amount (in this case, $100,000 per year as an annuity) to provide for their comfortable retirement. If the superannuant died before using up their allotted $1.5 million, the balance could be transferred to the superannuation fund of their dependents. An old-age pension would help those who live beyond 85. Thus the government would not be required to come to the aid of a person who should never have become a pauper in the first place.

6. In order to start the government superannuation fund, there is no need to raid present private funds. However, people could transfer whatever funds they have in their private funds to the government fund (up to the set limit).

Such government control of superannuation would:

a) guarantee every person a comfortable retirement income
b) save the costs of fund managers and prevent the fraudulent diversion of funds
c) provide funds for much-needed infrastructure development
d) ultimately decrease the general tax burden on the community and
e) release housing stock that is presently being held by investors to guarantee their retirement income.

From what we have said above, we must always consider the consequences of any particular change that occurs as part of the plan

I have extended the discussion of the health system into fields that appear unrelated. But finance for health is not quarantined. If health is to get a greater share of government revenue, then some other area must suffer. In order to analyze the overall situation, we need to look at the global structure of government finance.

In essence, governments have no money of their own—what they spend they must first derive from taxpayers. Hence, we need to consider *revenue as well as outlays*.

Diverting superannuation money from the private sector to the government would increase the availability of finance to the government. It would also decrease the amount of tax deductibility by limiting the nest egg that any individual may accumulate. The present system of allowing the limitless expansion of superannuation funds with concessional tax deductibility creates a distortion of the taxation system. This may not be a popular suggestion, but there is presently over a trillion dollars in superannuation funds that could be used more efficiently in the economy.

In respect to government outlays, I have suggested a number of mechanisms to decrease wastage and to decrease government liability.

Many of the problems of our present health system come about because very few understand the inter-relationships of government, hospital administration and medical personnel. Nor do many understand the games being played in each of these sectors. Hopefully, this book will help everyone understand the reason behind the games and costs. A sympathetic consideration of the needs and objectives of all of the players would be most helpful.

IN|DEX

www.ingramcontent.com/pod-product-compliance
Lightning Source LLC
Chambersburg PA
CBHW070906280326
41934CB00008B/1610